HEY, LET'S TALK

PUBERTY
WORKBOOK

HELPING **YOU** SURVIVE PUBERTY AND ALL
THE NEW REALITIES OF YOUR CHANGING BODY.

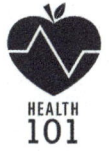

HEALTH 101 CURRICULUM

EMILY KISZKA, MA, BS, HEALTH EDUCATION

HEY, LET'S TALK!

Copyright © 2024 by Emily Kiszka

Published in the United States by: Health 101, LLC.

Content Production and Design: Emily Kiszka

All rights reserved. No part of this book may be reproduced by any mechanical, photographic, or electronic means, or in the form of a phonographic recording; nor may it be stored in a retrieval system, transmitted, or otherwise be copied for public or private use without prior written permission of the publisher.

The author of this workbook does not dispense medical advice or prescribe the use of any technique as a form of treatment for physical, emotional, or medical problems without the advice of a physician, either directly or indirectly. The intent of the author is only to offer information of a general nature to help in the quest for overall wellbeing. In the event the reader uses any information for personal reasons, the author and the publisher assume no responsibility.

Workbook ISBN (US): 979-8-89372-312-0

10 9 8 7 6 5 4 3 2 1

1st edition, 2024
Printed in the United States of America

HEY, LET'S TALK!

Check it off

WARM UP 2-5

Welcome Letter, Introduce Yourself, My Self-Portrait, More About Me

GETTING STARTED 6-12

Puberty Defined, Myth or Fact, Puberty Feelings, Whatcha Think?, Straight Talk, Puberty Maze

IT'S STILL THE SAME YOU 13-17

It's Still You, Heart Qualities, High Five To You, Color Me Beautiful, Mystery Message

ALL THE DETAILS 18-47

Word Identification, Word Search, Questions, Hmmm..., Identification, Let's Talk, Big Differences, Reminders, Rate Your Understanding, Myth or Fact

YOU AND YOUR LIFE 48-52

Times of Change, What Would You Do?, Puberty + Stress, Life Goals, Gratitude

ANONYMOUS QUESTIONS ....

JOURNAL PAPER ....

APPENDIX + GLOSSARY ....

HEALTH 101 | PAGE 1

HEY, LET'S TALK!

Welcome to "Hey, Let's Talk"- A personalized time of learning and exploration created just for you.

Together we will work through the topic of puberty and all the changes that come along in life as we get older.

Let's dive into all of your questions, all of the feelings, and all of the details! After we do, we will land in a comfortable spot where you can proudly stand tall and smile!

It's so great you're here!

HEY, LET'S TALK!

ooooooooooooooooooo

THIS WORKBOOK BELONGS TO:

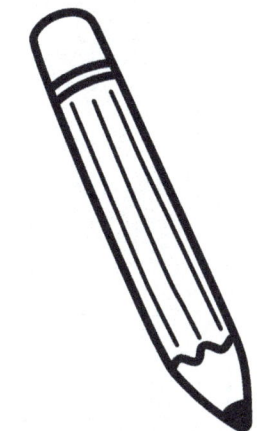

_____

ooooooooooooooooooo

HEALTH 101 | PAGE 3

HEY, LET'S TALK!

My Self-Portrait

DRAW A PICTURE OF YOURSELF × 3

What did you look like when you were little? What do you look like now?
What do you think you might look like in the future?

PAST **PRESENT** **FUTURE**

HEY, LET'S TALK!

More About Me

SHARE ALL OF YOUR FAVORITES!

There's so much to know about you. Will you share some of your favorite things below?

- **FAVORITE SEASON**
  or time of year

- **FAVORITE COLOR**
  or shade

- **FAVORITE ANIMAL**
  or character

- **FAVORITE ACTIVITY**
  or way to move your body

- **FAVORITE HOBBY**
  or free-time activity

- **FAVORITE SNACK**
  or beverage

HEALTH 101 | PAGE 5

HEY, LET'S TALK!

Puberty Defined

 Pu·ber·ty: the process of physical changes in the body that turn a child's body into an adult body.

Puberty is a big word for an even bigger time in life. During this time, your child body slowly starts turning into an adult body. These changes do not happen overnight. Just like your body has changed slowly since you were a baby, these changes happen slowly too.

As **puberty** is happening, we experience changes in our body, mind, and even in our feelings. You can see and feel some of those changes taking place, while other changes are not very noticeable because they take place slowly or even on the inside of your body.

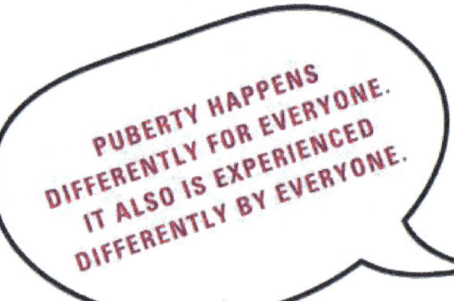

PUBERTY HAPPENS DIFFERENTLY FOR EVERYONE. IT ALSO IS EXPERIENCED DIFFERENTLY BY EVERYONE.

There can be all sorts of differences we experience in our personal journeys through **puberty**. It will always look a little different for every girl.

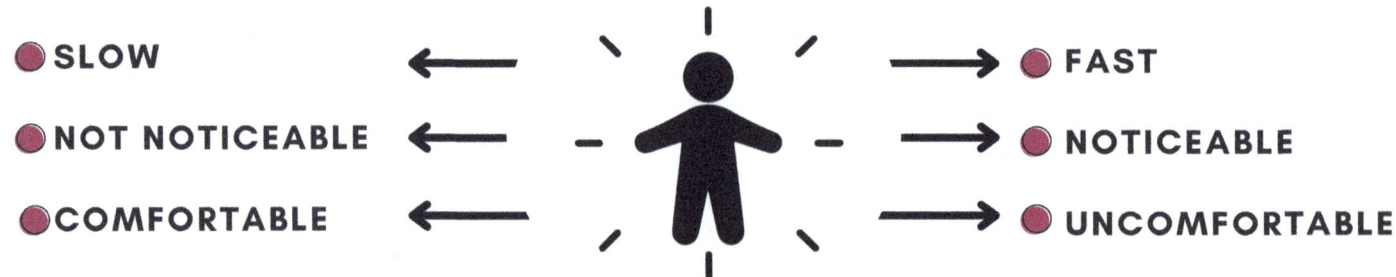

- SLOW ← → FAST
- NOT NOTICEABLE ← → NOTICEABLE
- COMFORTABLE ← → UNCOMFORTABLE

HEALTH 101 | PAGE 6

HEY, LET'S TALK!

MYTH OR FACT?

Make a guess by circling **MYTH OR FACT** for each of the statements below.

SITUATION	MYTH OR FACT?
• Puberty looks the same for girls as it does for boys.	MYTH OR FACT
• Everyone starts puberty at the same time.	MYTH OR FACT
• Everyone has happy feelings about going through puberty.	MYTH OR FACT
• Hormones are the cause of changes in puberty.	MYTH OR FACT
• There are things you can do to slow down puberty.	MYTH OR FACT
• People can always tell when you are going through puberty.	MYTH OR FACT
• Your feelings and emotions can feel different during puberty.	MYTH OR FACT
• Some parts of puberty can feel uncomfortable.	MYTH OR FACT
• Puberty happens slowly, spanning a few years.	MYTH OR FACT
• Puberty is an important part of your life.	MYTH OR FACT

HEY, LET'S TALK!

Puberty Feelings

 Feel·ings: an emotional state or reaction.

Puberty comes with a lot of change! Change of any kind can bring about **feelings** for us. Sometimes change can feel difficult or scary, while other times it can feel exciting and joyful.

It might surprise you to hear this, but your **feelings** toward the changes you notice in puberty are normal. It's true! It is okay to not like the changes you are seeing in your body. Or, perhaps you don't feel that way at all. Maybe you feel proud and happy about some of the changes. There are no wrong **feelings**.

Sometimes in life, we can experience a mix of different **feelings** at the same time. And that's okay too! You are allowed to think and feel any way you want to. All **feelings** you might have about puberty are understandable and acceptable.

You also don't have to be alone with your **feelings** about puberty. It's important to find a safe adult with whom you can share your **feelings** and questions.

Just remember that since the beginning of time, girls have gone through puberty. Your mom, your grandmother, the lady down the street, and so on. Take comfort in knowing that you are surrounded by women who have been through the very same things you are experiencing.

> EVERYONE EXPERIENCES DIFFERENT FEELINGS ABOUT THIS TIME IN LIFE. SOME GIRLS MIGHT NOT LIKE THE CHANGES WHILE OTHERS MIGHT FEEL EXCITED ABOUT THEM!

HEALTH 101 | PAGE 8

HEY, LET'S TALK!

WHATCHA THINK?

Circle all the feelings you feel about puberty.
Any feelings that you are feeling are perfectly normal.

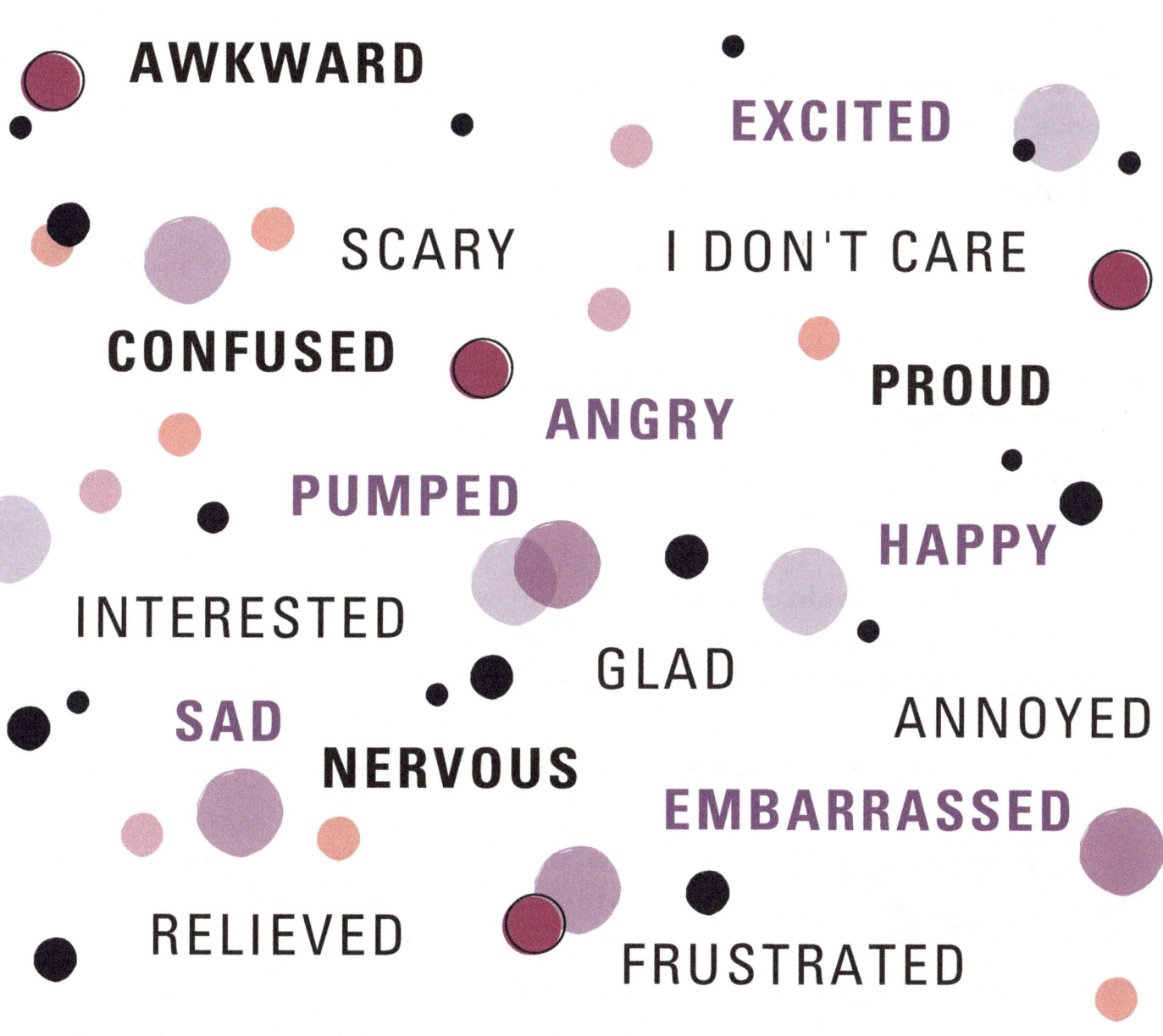

AWKWARD

EXCITED

SCARY   I DON'T CARE

CONFUSED
              ANGRY   **PROUD**
       PUMPED
                          HAPPY
INTERESTED
              GLAD
    SAD   ANNOYED
       NERVOUS
                  EMBARRASSED

  RELIEVED
              FRUSTRATED

ANY OTHER FEELINGS? _____

HEALTH 101 | PAGE 9

HEY, LET'S TALK!

Straight Talk

Does the topic of puberty feel weird or awkward to you? If so, you're not alone! Here are thoughts and feelings shared by high school girls as they look back on when they went through puberty.

- "**I wish** someone told me everything about puberty so that I didn't have to Google stuff."

- "**I wish** talking about this stuff wasn't so weird."

- "**Other people** going through puberty feel uncomfortable in their body too, they just may not show it."

- "We all end up on the other side of puberty as adults. But it seriously **does not matter** one bit how slow or fast you go through it."

- "**I wish** someone told me how to take care of myself in all the different ways once puberty hits."

- "Looking back I realize so much of what was talked about by other students was **wrong**. So many kids have no idea what they are even talking about even though they sound like they know it all."

- "I know it seems gross, but just **try your best** to roll with it."

- "**I wish** my parents talked to me in more detail abaut all this stuff."

- "**I wish** someone told me how my first period would be- with all the details I need to know."

HEALTH 101 | PAGE 10

HEY, LET'S TALK!

" I JUST WISH I COULD ASSURE YOUNGER GIRLS THAT LIFE GETS BETTER."

HEY, LET'S TALK!

It's a maze...

BUT YOU'VE GOT THIS!

PUBERTY can feel like a maze at times, with lots of turns and dead ends, but you will *always* make it through to the other side!

CAN YOU MAKE YOUR WAY THROUGH THIS MAZE?

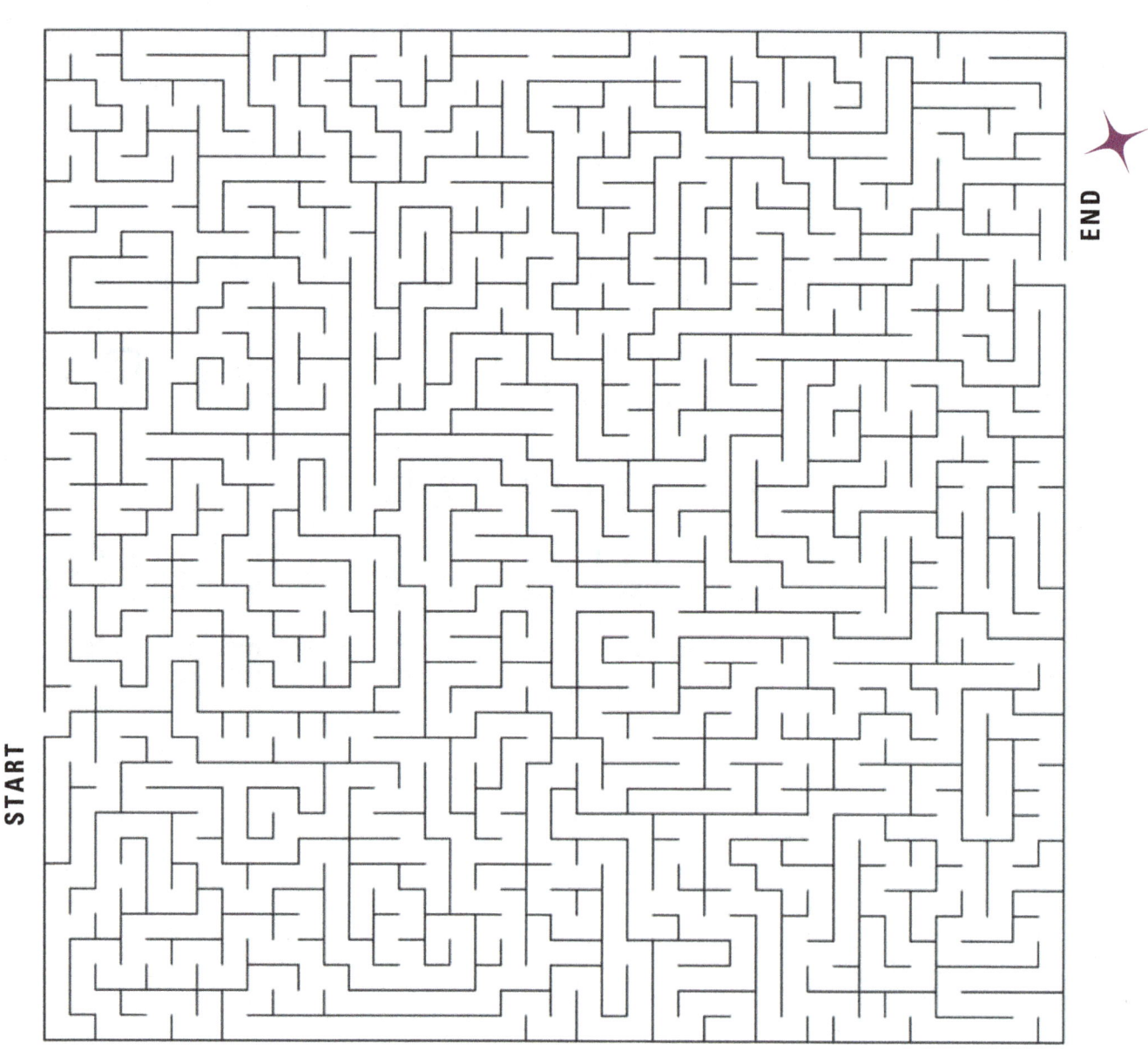

HEALTH 101 | PAGE 12

HEY, LET'S TALK!

It's Still You

 You: special and valuable since the day you were born!

All of the changes and feelings that happen during puberty can leave you feeling confused. Sometimes you might feel like you are becoming someone different, or perhaps like you are leaving a part of yourself behind.

But take comfort in this: although your body might be changing in different ways on the outside, you are still the very same **you** on the inside!

Even though your body changes, your value and worth does not. **You** are just as special as you were the day you were created, and **you will be valuable forever**.

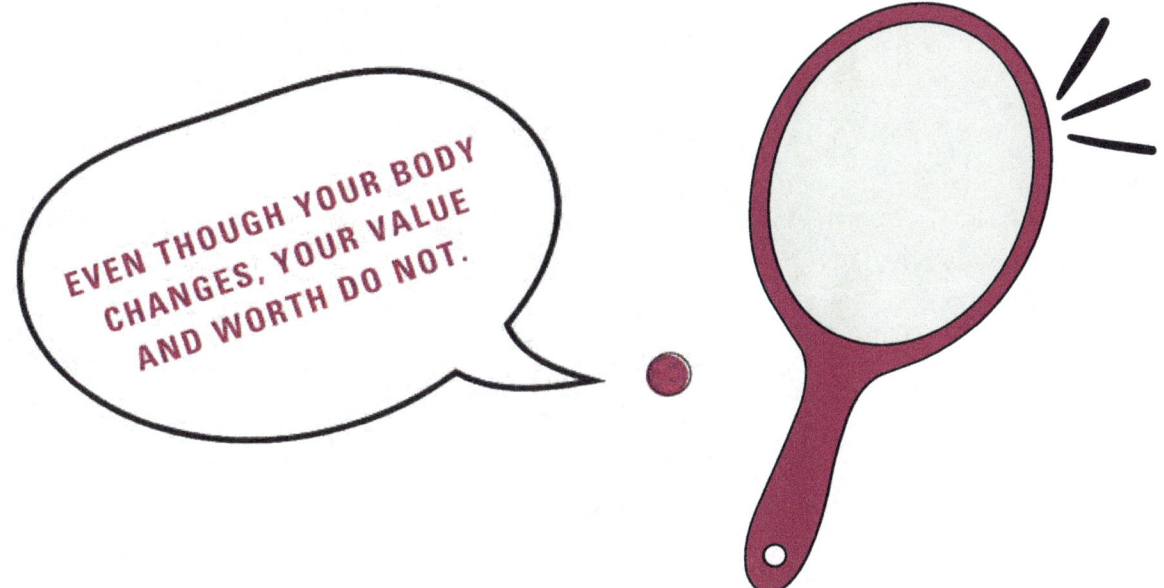

HEALTH 101 | PAGE 13

HEY, LET'S TALK!

Heart Qualities

Circle words from this list that are qualities of **YOUR** heart. Write them down in the hand on the next page.

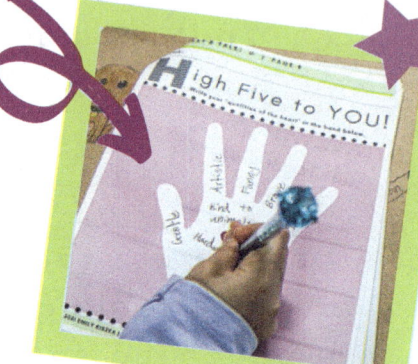

- Kind
- Includes others
- Kind to animals
- Shares
- Great memory
- Fun
- Has great ideas
- Great Planner
- Organized
- Trustworthy
- Respectful
- Brave
- Funny
- Truthful
- Artistic
- Inspirational
- Helper
- Gentle
- Good Leader
- Safe friend
- Rescuer
- Good listener
- Protective
- Loving
- Quick
- Patient
- Joyful

- Easy to talk to
- Fair
- Hard Worker
- Wise
- Peaceful
- Silly
- Energetic
- Thoughtful
- Adventurous
- Interesting
- Entertaining
- Strong
- Positive
- Optimistic
- Sweet
- Creative
- Smart
- Gives good advice
- Logical
- Impressive
- Reliable
- Mature
- Dreamer
- Helps little kids
- Sensitive
- Accepting
- Capable

- Nice
- Routined
- Proud
- Caring
- Understanding
- Inquisitive
- Professional
- Calm
- Exciting
- Talkative
- Deep Thinker
- Loyal
- Good Communicator
- Perceptive
- Motivated
- Assertive
- Compassionate
- Forgiving
- Consistent
- Appreciative

HEALTH 101 | PAGE 14

HEY, LET'S TALK!

HIGH FIVE TO YOU!
Write your **"qualities of the heart"** in or around the hand below.

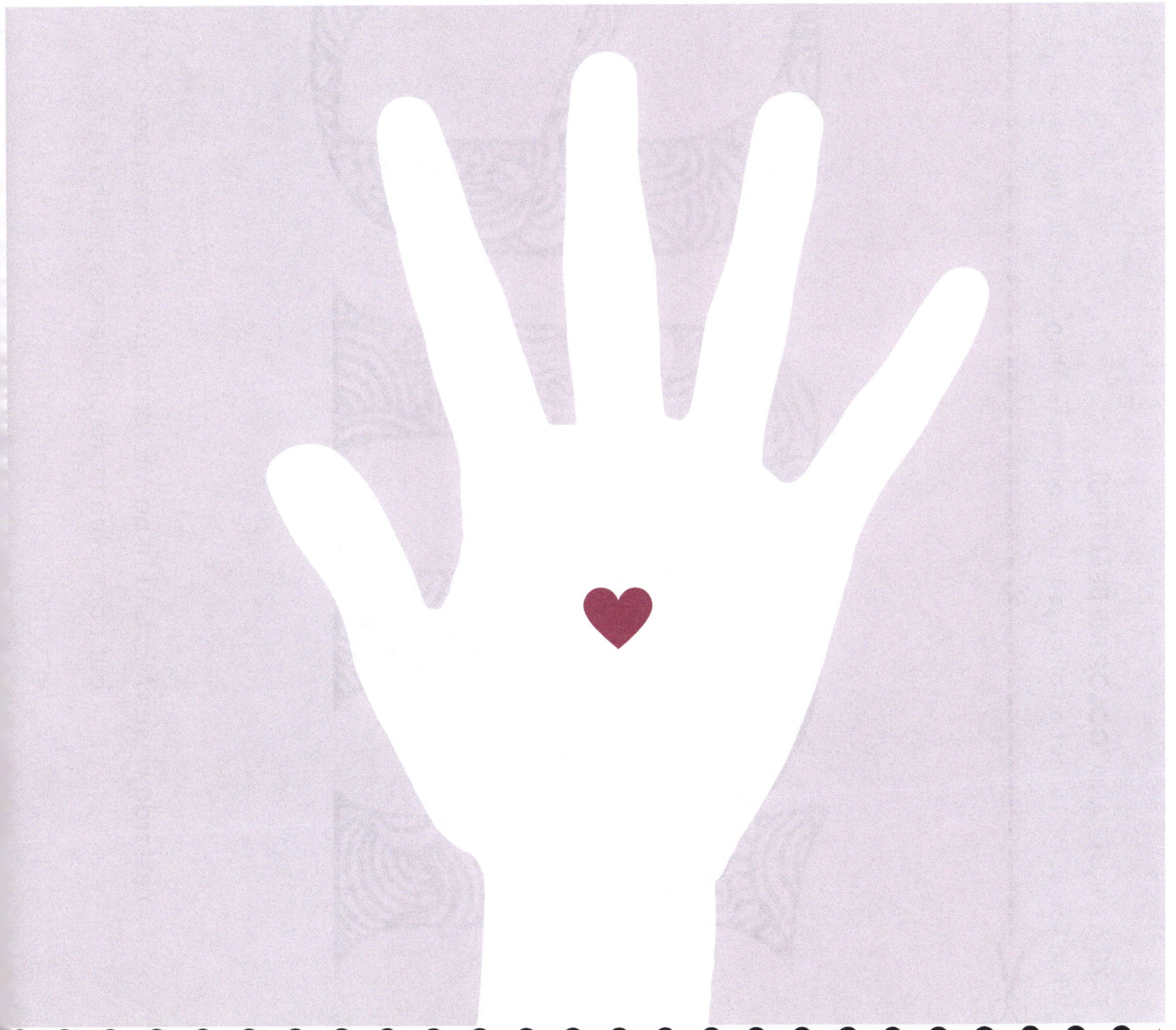

HEALTH 101 | PAGE 15

HEY, LET'S TALK!

TAKE A MINUTE AND "COLOR ME BEAUTIFUL."
While you color, reflect on all of your awesomeness. Then cut it out and keep it if you'd like!

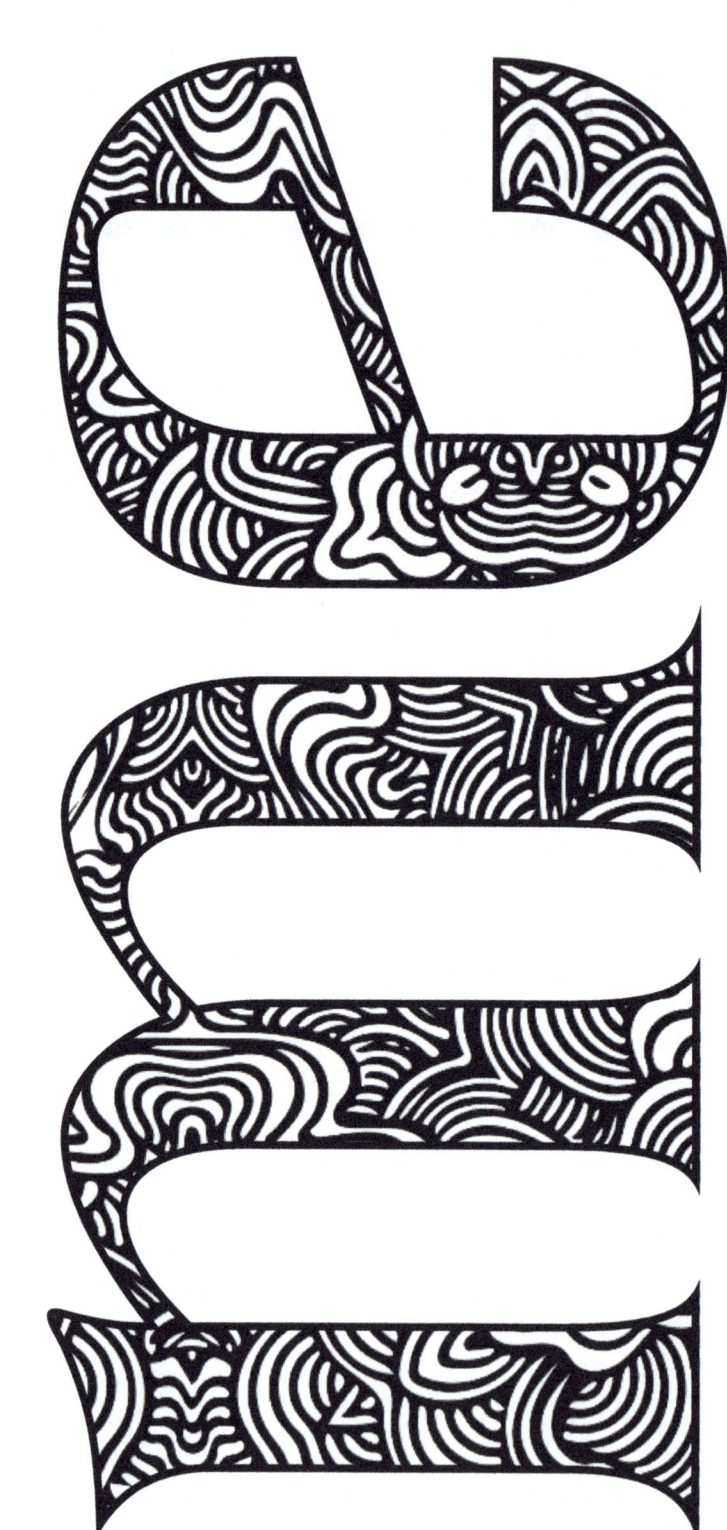

Yesterday I was ME, and I'll be ME tomorrow. This time does not change ME, but adds even more uniqueness to who I am.

HEALTH 101 | PAGE 16

HEY, LET'S TALK!

Mystery Message

1. **Find** all the words on the list.
2. **Copy** the unused letters starting at the top left corner into the blanks to reveal the hidden message.

Words can go in any direction and can cross over each other.

```
S E I T I L A U Q M Y B O U N
W I L N L S S T T A I O L L O
B E T H E E E S A T M D E S I
D P E L C E I A L U Y Y O U T
O L F E N N T T H R E O T H A
E R I A L S I E P E D E O F M
P U G H B K E R R U T Y E L R
S E B J C T R W I P B U G U O
R G G S E G N A H C Q E M F F
E Y N R T M U M P I Z R R I N
C Y R I O B Y O N S D J V T I
L I F E L W I U L O D J I U Y
G Z S K J E I U A T B E E A R
I P O H C T E N M A H J K E M
K V P N W N R F G E N C E B K
```

Beautiful Body   Changes
Child   Feelings   Growing
Information Life   Mature
Preteen   Puberty   Qualities
Self   Sparkle   Teenager
Unique

HIDDEN MESSAGE ABOUT YOU:

_ _ _ _ _ _ _ _ _ _ _ _ _ _ _

_ _ _ _ _ _ _ _ _ _ _ _ _ _ _

_ _ _ _ _ _ _ _ _ _ _ _ _ _ _

_ _ _ _ _ _ _ _ _ _ _ _ _ _ _

HEALTH 101 | PAGE 17

HEY, LET'S TALK!

WORDS WORDS WORDS

DIRECTIONS: (Circle) all of the words you **can** define.

Underline any of the words you **cannot** define.

- PERIOD
- BREAST
- MENSTRUAL CYCLE
- HORMONES
- CHANGES
- BRA
- PAD
- VAGINA
- MOOD
- RAZOR
- WEIGHT
- BOOBS
- CONFIDENCE
- UTERUS

- PUBIC HAIR
- EMOTIONS
- HYGIENE
- FEELINGS
- SHAVE
- TAMPON
- BIKINI LINE
- DEODORANT
- ACNE
- PANTY LINER
- HEIGHT
- BREAST BUD
- GROWTH SPURT
- DISCHARGE

HEY, LET'S TALK!

Find the Words

```
p t f b p v m p h e j e s s r
t u a j r i c o d u j l e n g
r h b m s k f s f a v q g o a
a b g i p u g t a p a d n i w
u j i i c o m u q n u t a t c
j j c h e h n r w g i g h o t
x p y q b w a e s r f g c m n
s t s a e r b i t o i w a e a
f e e l i n g s r w v i a v r
a g u y j w d r c i s r d h o
p u b e r t y o h n b o e z d
h o r m o n e s o g o i a y o
w n f e v a h s t m g c l y e
n e g o r t s e r h n k h c d
e r u t s o p r t e a b s b s
```

Acne
Changes
Estrogen
Height
Pad
Puberty
Tampon

Bra
Deodorant
Feelings
Hormones
Posture
Pubichair
Vagina

Breasts
Emotions
Growing
Mood
Posture
Shave
Weight

HEALTH 101 | PAGE 19

HEY, LET'S TALK!

QUESTIONS?

The topic of puberty brings up a lot of **thoughts and questions**. List some questions you have or are wondering about in the box below.

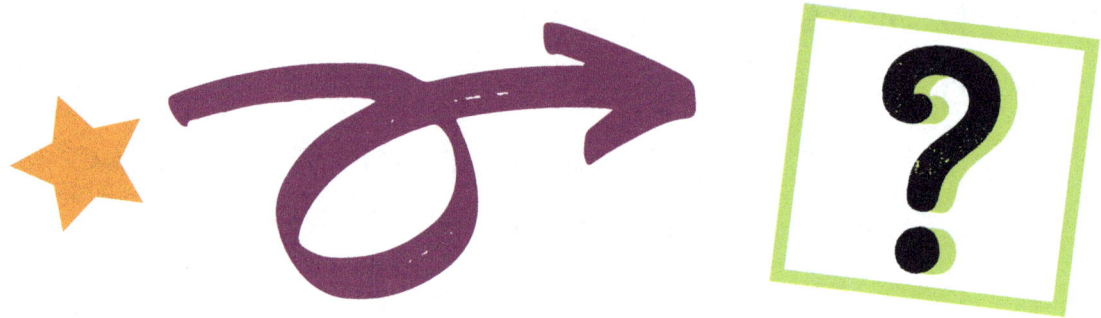

Is it true that...   Why is it that...   What happens when...   I'm wondering if...

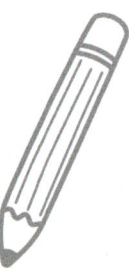

HEY, LET'S TALK!

Hmmmm......

Who are the "safe" people in your life? Brainstorm a list in the circle below.

🔊 A **"safe"** person to talk to is someone in your life who makes sure to keep you protected physically and who cares for you emotionally, too. You trust that they will have helpful advice that benefits you in life.

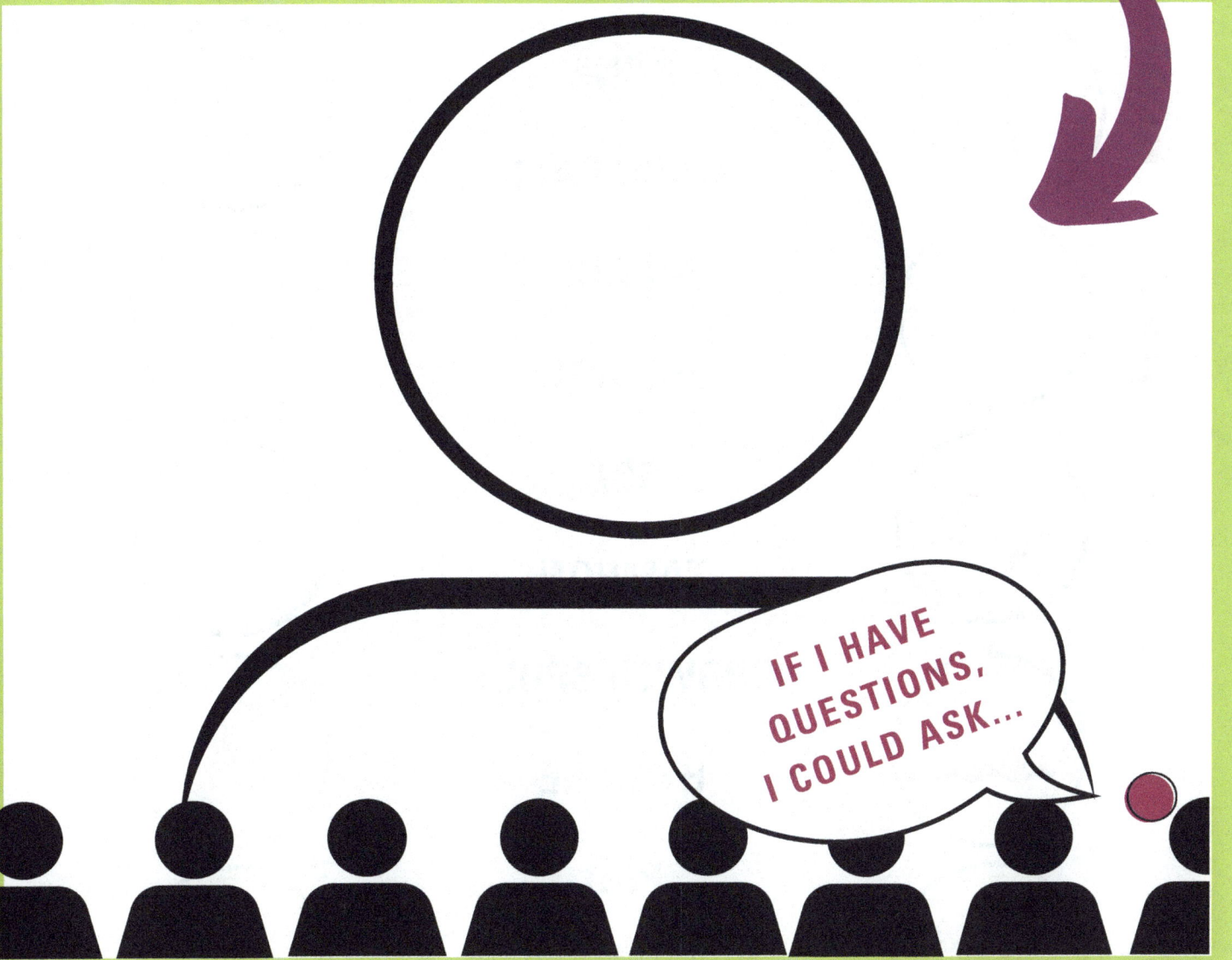

HEALTH 101 | PAGE 21

HEY, LET'S TALK!

Identification

Can you **draw a line** connecting the puberty term to the matching picture?

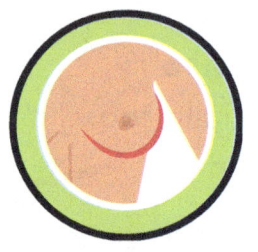

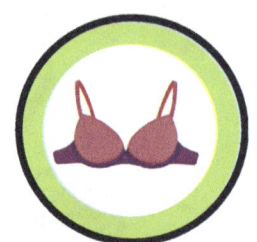
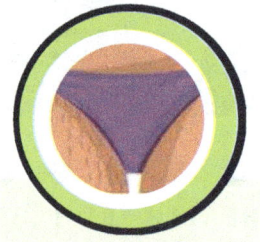

DEODORANT

RAZOR

ACNE

PUBIC HAIR

MOODS

BREAST

BRA

TAMPON

GROWTH SPURT

HYGIENE

PAD

PERIOD

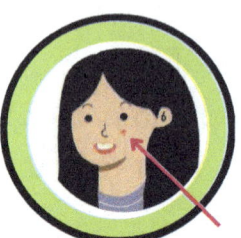
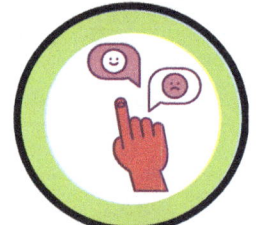

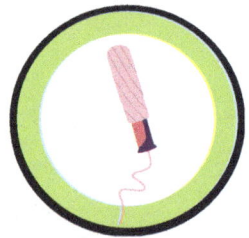
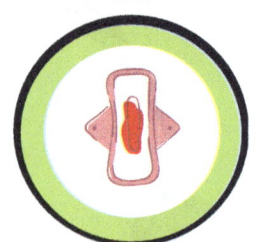
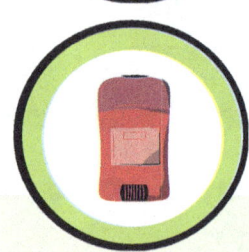

HEALTH 101 | PAGE 22

HEY, LET'S TALK!

Let's talk...

Let's explore all of the information from pages **24-43**. Each topic will have some helpful information for you, as well as some little tips and interesting facts! Complete the worksheet that goes with each topic and be sure to write down questions you have along the way.

Information organized by topic!

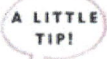

Check-in page for every topic!

HEALTH 101 | PAGE 23

HEY, LET'S TALK!

FACT SHEET

COMPLETE THIS WORKSHEET USING THE FACT POSTER.

✉ **TOPIC:** MOOD SWINGS

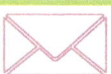 **EXPLANATION:**

Hormones increase in our bodies as we enter puberty. The main hormone for females is called estrogen. Estrogen is the "invisible force" behind all the changes you see and feel in your body. You may notice that things feel more upsetting, frustrating, or worrisome than they ever used to. On the flip side, even excitement feels more exciting. You're probably familiar with different moods, but thanks to estrogen, you're seeing a lot more moods than you have in previous years, and those moods might feel bigger and stronger than you remember. This can be hard for you and your friends and family, but it is completely normal.

Something important to know, however, is that all feelings are valid. Feelings are temporary. Give yourself time and space to experience your feelings and work through them. You also never have to be alone with your feelings. It is important to find a trusted person to share your feelings and thoughts with. This could be a parent, teacher, counselor, mentor, or close friend.

Feelings of attraction for the opposite sex can also start to occur. This could feel confusing or strange. You can blame these different feelings on hormones too! That's what causes feelings to be different than when you were little.
But that doesn't mean anything has to change. You are still in control of all of your decisions and life choices.

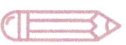 **DID YOU KNOW?**

Deep breaths can help.
Try finding a quiet place and do 10 nice and slow deep breaths.

In through your nose and out through your mouth. It won't take all your problems away, but it will take some of the "sting" out of those tough-to-manage feelings!

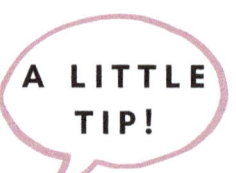

A LITTLE TIP!

HEALTH 101 | PAGE 24

HEY, LET'S TALK!

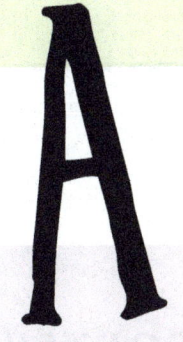ll the details

USE THE FACT SHEET TO COMPLETE THE BOXES BELOW.

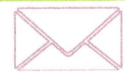 **TOPIC:** MOOD SWINGS

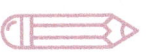 **THINGS TO REMEMBER:**
-
-
-
-
-

 I'M WONDERING:
-
-

 CHECK IN:

Moods feel stronger during puberty because of:

a. hormones
b. unnatural body changes
c. poor sleeping habits

HEALTH 101 | PAGE 25

HEY, LET'S TALK!

Fact Sheet

COMPLETE THIS WORKSHEET USING THE FACT POSTER.

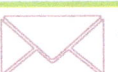 **TOPIC:** GROWING

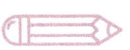 **EXPLANATION:**

During puberty, your body will go through some periods of fast growth. This is known as a "growth spurt." You might notice that you're getting taller, stronger, and faster. These changes occur because your "child body" is slowly turning into your "adult body." In order for your body to do its best as it moves through life, you may notice that changes such as your hips widening and some weight gain occurs. Just like we can't do anything to keep our body from growing, we can't do anything to slow down puberty changes either.

Other changes in your body during this time could include acne on your face and/or body. Acne is made up of pimples, which are red, irritated bumps on your skin. It's important to wash your face every day with a gentle facial cleanser, although it's important to know that acne can't always be prevented. You can talk to your doctor if acne starts to become a very big issue for you.

Did you know that boys experience changes during puberty too? They do! But puberty looks very different for them. Changes they experience include a deepening voice, bigger shoulders, and a faster growing rate. The hormone they have in their body that's behind all of these different changes is called "testosterone."

 **DID YOU KNOW?**

You might notice pains in your legs at bedtime when they are growing at a faster speed than usual. In fact, you may have noticed this as a young child too. It can be difficult to go to sleep when your legs hurt. Using a heating pad on them can help or you can rub them with lotion or leg cramp ointment. If the pain is a big issue for you, you can talk to an adult about possibly using some pain relief medicine, or seeing your doctor".

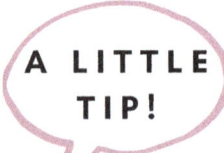 A LITTLE TIP!

HEY, LET'S TALK!

All the Details

USE THE FACT SHEET TO COMPLETE THE BOXES BELOW.

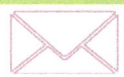 **TOPIC:** GROWING

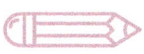 **THINGS TO REMEMBER:**

-
-
-
-
-

 I'M WONDERING:

-
-

 CHECK IN:

The main female hormone behind growing changes is:

a. testosterone
b. estrogen
c. influenza

HEALTH 101 | PAGE 27

HEY, LET'S TALK!

FACT SHEET

COMPLETE THIS WORKSHEET USING THE FACT POSTER.

TOPIC: SMELLING AWESOME

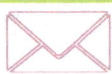
EXPLANATION:

It's important to smell awesome! Well, at least we don't want to smell bad, right? Unlike when you were little, your body will need a lot more hygiene habits. There are things we have to do in order to ensure we don't have offensive body odor. A lot of pre-teens and teenagers think using sprays and perfumes will be a sure way to not smell bad, but in reality, all that does is cover up odor, not eliminate it. You can use a body spray, but first you have to make sure you are squeaky clean.

In order to prevent unpleasant smells, you will need to do a few things:
-Wear deodorant in your armpits.
-Shower every day.
-Wash your clothes after each wear.
-Change your bed sheets at least 2 times a month.
-Wash your hair more often and scrub your scalp.
-Keep up good mouth care: Brush teeth, floss, use mouthwash.

If using soap in and around your genitals causes irritation, itchiness, or dryness, you could get a special wash for that area. There are shower cleansing washes that help regulate your natural PH and are a great idea to consider if regular soaps or body shower gels cause irritation.

DID YOU KNOW?

There is a great secret to avoiding bad breath. It's your tongue! Most bad breath comes from your tongue, not your teeth! So when you are brushing your teeth, don't forget to brush your tongue, too! In the toothbrush aisle, you will find "**tongue scrapers.**"

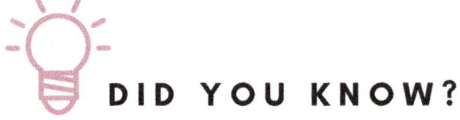

HEALTH 101 | PAGE 28

HEY, LET'S TALK!

All the Details

USE THE FACT SHEET TO COMPLETE THE BOXES BELOW.

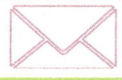 **TOPIC:** SMELLING AWESOME

 **THINGS TO REMEMBER:**

-
-
-
-
-

 I'M WONDERING:

-
-

 CHECK IN:

Bad breath primarily comes from smelly bacteria that lives:

a. on your teeth
b. in your throat
c. on your tongue

HEALTH 101 | PAGE 29

HEY, LET'S TALK!

FACT SHEET

COMPLETE THIS WORKSHEET USING THE FACT POSTER.

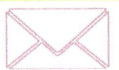 **TOPIC:** HAIR

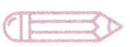 **EXPLANATION:**

When your hormones start to increase, you will start to notice changes in body hair. Your leg hair will be more noticeable and you'll get darker and coarser hair in other places. These areas include your armpits and your pubic region (this hair is known as pubic hair). The pubic region is right around where a zipper on your pants would be, all the way out to the crease where your leg meets your body (see **Appendix A**).

Your armpits and pubic region contain very helpful, germ fighting glands underneath the skin. These glands protect you from a lot of harmful things that enter your body through the air, food, drink, and more! That makes those areas on your body very important. The new thicker and darker hair in these areas appears to help protect these areas and keep us healthy every day.

Commonly, girls will shave the very top part of their leg where their bathing suit or underwear crease is. This is commonly known as the "bikini line." It's up to you whether you'd like to shave or trim the hair that grows in this area. You can shave, trim, or wax any of it or leave the hair there entirely alone.

 **DID YOU KNOW?**

Pubic hair is curly and sometimes it can get trapped under the skin causing a little painful bump.

This is known as an ingrown hair. You can do a little gentle exfoliating with a washcloth or gentle scrub when you're in the shower to help prevent this. They do go away after a little while.

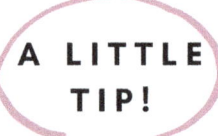 **A LITTLE TIP!**

HEALTH 101 | PAGE 30

HEY, LET'S TALK!

All the Details

USE THE FACT SHEET TO COMPLETE THE BOXES BELOW.

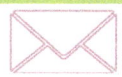 **TOPIC:** HAIR

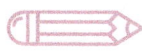 **THINGS TO REMEMBER:**

-
-
-
-
-

 I'M WONDERING:

-
-

 CHECK IN:

Pubic hair is your body's attempt to create a barrier to protect:

a. your body temperature
b. germ-fighting glands
c. body odor

HEALTH 101 | PAGE 31

HEY, LET'S TALK!

FACT SHEET

COMPLETE THIS WORKSHEET USING THE FACT POSTER.

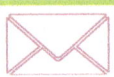 **TOPIC:** SHAVING

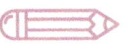 **EXPLANATION:**

Shaving is something a lot of girls choose to do as they get older. The areas most commonly shaved are legs and armpits. In order to avoid discomfort, it's important to use a sharp razor, water, and soap or shaving cream.

You can use soap instead of buying fancy shaving cream and it will work just as well- if not better! As long as the area you're shaving is wet and slippery, you should be good to go! Hair will grow back within a few days.

The age when you start shaving is different for everyone. For some, it's when hair seems more coarse, dark, or noticeable. There's nothing wrong with shaving or not shaving! In fact, in certain cultures around the world, shaving is not the norm for women. Just remember, although it might seem exciting at first, shaving quickly becomes another thing on your to-do list, like making your bed. Just like a made bed, it looks nice and feels nice, but there is upkeep!

Razors can cause razor burn if you shave the same spot too many times. Razor burn looks like red bumps and it hurts! Sometimes your skin might need a day or two break from shaving.

When shopping, you will see razors that are marketed to men, some to women.

It doesn't matter which you use, as long as it is a good quality product and gives you a comfortable shaving experience.

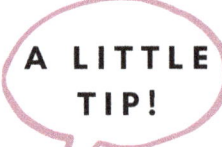
A LITTLE TIP!

HEALTH 101 | PAGE 32

HEY, LET'S TALK!

All the Details

USE THE FACT SHEET TO COMPLETE THE BOXES BELOW.

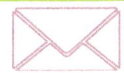 **TOPIC:** SHAVING

 **THINGS TO REMEMBER:**

-
-
-
-
-

 I'M WONDERING:

-
-

 CHECK IN:

In order to avoid discomfort, it's important to make sure the area you're **shaving** is (choose one):

a. hairy
b. wet
c. cold

HEALTH 101 | PAGE 33

HEY, LET'S TALK!

FACT SHEET

COMPLETE THIS WORKSHEET USING THE FACT POSTER.

✉ **TOPIC:** BREASTS

✏ **EXPLANATION:**

Breasts start to show up as a tiny little bump or puff under your nipple on your chest. These are "breast buds." They will feel painful at times, especially if they are bumped or pressed. Although that sounds like a real "pain," know that it is completely normal. They hurt because they are getting ready to grow. In fact, breasts are often very tender until they are done growing.

Speaking of growing, breasts will continue to grow through your middle and high school years and will stop around the age of eighteen, sometimes sooner (see **Appendix B**). Breasts come in all shapes and sizes. Breasts can change size in life based on other factors such as weight gain or loss, pregnancy, and menstrual cycles (period). Each month, during the period, some girls may notice that their breasts are a little more tender, while other girls may not notice it at all.

It may be hard to believe, but boys can get breast buds too. Breast buds can show up for them around the same age, and often a little closer to middle school or high school years. Similarly, it appears as a small bump under the nipple that is tender to the touch. The difference is that boys have a different hormone, testosterone, which will cause this bump to go away and flatten out as they get older.

💡 **DID YOU KNOW?**

When it comes to bras, every girl is different. Some may want a traditional, slightly padded bra, while others may be excited about a fun looking one with cups that provide more support. Some girls may hate the idea of a bra. That's perfectly normal too! One of the best suggestions in that case is to try a sports bra. Sports bras come in all shapes and colors.

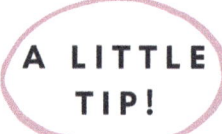 **A LITTLE TIP!** Wearing one is not much different than how your bathing suit feels. Again, up to you!

HEALTH 101 | PAGE 34

HEY, LET'S TALK!

All the Details

USE THE FACT SHEET TO COMPLETE THE BOXES BELOW.

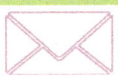 **TOPIC:** BREASTS

 **THINGS TO REMEMBER:**
-
-
-
-
-

 I'M WONDERING:
-
-

 CHECK IN:

When breasts are growing, they can feel:

a. extra hard
b. hot to the touch
c. painful when bumped

HEALTH 101 | PAGE 35

HEY, LET'S TALK!

Fact Sheet

COMPLETE THIS WORKSHEET USING THE FACT POSTER.

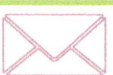 **TOPIC:** DISCHARGE

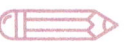 **EXPLANATION:**

Early on in puberty, usually between third and sixth grade, you may start to notice a small amount of wetness in your underwear when you are just going about your day. This isn't "pee," as I'm sure you know. But if it's not urine, then what is it? This wetness is called discharge. Discharge is intended to leave your body every day through the vagina. The vagina (see **Appendix D**) is an opening located between your urethra (where urine leaves your body) and your anus (where poop leaves your body). Since you aren't supposed to wash the inside of the vagina, your body has a way of doing it for you- and that's discharge. You know what other part of your body does this? Here's a clue: it's another delicate part of your body that you are not supposed to wash with soap. Your eye! Your eye is cleaned every night when you sleep, which is why you wake up with a little bit of crust or "sleep" in your eye in the morning. It's this same cleansing process that occurs in the vagina. This tiny bit of fluid leaving your body cleans your vagina.

Even though discharge might feel uncomfortable at first, you will not notice it after a while. Once your body is used to this new occurrence, you will hardly notice it's happening and it will not feel bothersome to you.

Don't be alarmed. Discharge is a sign that your body is working properly! Discharge can appear white, clear, or even off-white. There shouldn't be any other colors associated with discharge, nor any pain or odor either. You can expect to notice discharge every day during the start of puberty all the way into adulthood.

 **DID YOU KNOW?**

If discharge does ever feel too bothersome to you, you can always use a "panty liner." Liners can be purchased at any grocery or drug store. They are tiny and thin. You stick one to your underwear each morning and can experience a dry feeling all day. You will hardly notice that the liner is there. They tear off easily and can get tossed in the trash. Easy peasy for any girl who prefers this option.

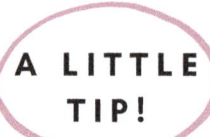 A LITTLE TIP!

HEALTH 101 | PAGE 36

HEY, LET'S TALK!

All the Details

USE THE FACT SHEET TO COMPLETE THE BOXES BELOW.

 **TOPIC:** DISCHARGE

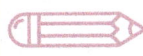 **THINGS TO REMEMBER:**

-
-
-
-
-

 I'M WONDERING:

-
-

 CHECK IN:

Discharge is a way for the vagina to clean itself, which is helpful because you shouldn't be cleaning inside your vagina with soap.

a. True
b. False

HEALTH 101 | PAGE 37

HEY, LET'S TALK!

FACT SHEET

COMPLETE THIS WORKSHEET USING THE FACT POSTER.

TOPIC: PERIODS

EXPLANATION:

At a certain point in puberty, you will start getting a period. A period, more appropriately known as a menstrual period, takes place once every month. During this particular week, blood leaves the body through the vagina a little at a time, over the course of days. Your vagina (see **Appendix D**) is an opening located between your urethra (where urine leaves your body) and your anus (where poop leaves your body). The blood that leaves your body during this time originates in your uterus (see **Appendix C**).

The uterus sends this blood out of your body during the period because your body does not need it. There is only a need for this blood when a woman is pregnant. Although our eyes see our period as "blood," our body, when pregnant, sees it as an important substance that surrounds, nourishes, and grows the baby. In pregnancy, the uterus becomes an amazing little home for a growing baby. The vagina, also known as the birth canal, leads the baby from the uterus into the world when the baby is born.

Since every girl is different, there are differences in period experiences too. Some girls might have a period that takes as little as 4 days while others have periods that can last for a week. Some struggle with a lot of cramps, while others may have minimal pain. Other differences can include the amount of blood flow, mood swings, cravings, and breast tenderness.

Your period will be unique to your body.

DID YOU KNOW?

Some girls assume that blood loss must hurt, but this isn't the case. The area where the blood is leaving the body is not a wound, it's an opening (your vagina). There may be cramping or discomfort in the uterus, however. If you need relief from cramps, you can use a heating pad or pain relief medicine. Research shows that it's helpful to keep your body moving with light exercise if you can. It may help the cramps.

A LITTLE TIP!

HEALTH 101 | PAGE 38

HEY, LET'S TALK!

All the Details

USE THE FACT SHEET TO COMPLETE THE BOXES BELOW.

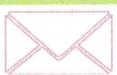 **TOPIC:** PERIODS

 **THINGS TO REMEMBER:**

-
-
-
-
-

 I'M WONDERING:

-
-

 CHECK IN:

During your period, blood leaves the body because you are:

a. pregnant
b. not pregnant
c. having a medical issue

HEALTH 101 | PAGE 39

HEY, LET'S TALK!

Fact Sheet

COMPLETE THIS WORKSHEET USING THE FACT POSTER.

✉ **TOPIC:** PERIOD SUPPLIES

✏ **EXPLANATION:**

There are a number of products you can buy to use when you have your period, all of which are designed differently to meet a wide variety of preferences and needs. There are pads, tampons, panty liners, diva cups, and even period underwear. These options are known as "Feminine Hygiene Products." All options come with different pros and cons so it's important for you to think about which options make you feel most comfortable.

A lot of girls have a mini-clutch or compartment of a purse or bag where they keep an emergency stash of period supplies in case of a period emergency. You could even consider designating a little hiding spot for these items in your family's car, so that they're with you whenever you travel. Even if you haven't gotten your period yet, you could talk to a trusted adult about getting these supplies in advance and having them ready at home for when you do need them. Also, many public bathrooms have pads and tampons to take or purchase when you're in need.

The days of your period usually correlate with how much blood flow you experience. The very first day and the last day (or two) usually have the smallest amount of blood. The largest amount of blood is typically experienced right in the middle portion of your period. Knowing this can help you plan ahead for what you need.

💡 **DID YOU KNOW?**

Did you know that once you've had your first period, you can get good at knowing when your next period is due? By looking at a calendar and counting out the weeks, you can tell when your next period will happen. The older you get, the more accurate this calendar-counting process becomes! See **Appendix E** for more information.

A LITTLE TIP!

HEALTH 101 | PAGE 40

HEY, LET'S TALK!

All the Details

USE THE FACT SHEET TO COMPLETE THE BOXES BELOW.

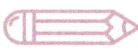 **TOPIC:** PERIOD SUPPLIES

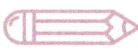 **THINGS TO REMEMBER:**

-
-
-
-
-

 I'M WONDERING:

-
-

 CHECK IN:

There are many different types of period supplies you can use, depending on what you consider:

a. comfortable
b. effective
c. both

HEALTH 101 | PAGE 41

HEY, LET'S TALK!

FACT SHEET

COMPLETE THIS WORKSHEET USING THE FACT POSTER.

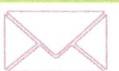 **TOPIC:** CONFIDENCE

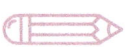 **EXPLANATION:**

With so many changes going on in your body, it can feel like you're facing a lot of uncertainty. Sometimes we may feel less confident when things look or feel different than they used to, or when we look or feel different from other kids around us. But it's important to remember that confidence comes from the inside and we can grow our confidence. Did you know that? It's true. Confidence doesn't always come naturally.

As you get older, you are faced with many new challenges that can leave you feeling unsure of your ability to handle it all. Often times, people wait for confidence to come to them before they try something new or make a brave move when they are feeling nervous. But it's the opposite. Confidence comes **after** bravery. You have to take brave steps, try new things, reach outside your normal comfort zone enough times, and the confidence will start to slowly build. It's a huge myth to believe that we need to wait for confidence to show up automatically. In a way, this is really encouraging to know. **You have the power to create your own level of confidence.**

You have an **internal voice**. It is how you speak to yourself. How you speak to yourself is developed over the course of your life. It's important for you to take a close look at your internal voice and inspect how it sounds. Are you criticizing or talking rudely to yourself? Try talking to yourself the way you would a best friend. Practice showing yourself kindness and understanding. The results will be huge for your confidence!

 **DID YOU KNOW?**

We can help ourselves show confidence by keeping a good posture with our body. Practice holding your shoulders up and back. Wear a smile when you can and do your best to maintain eye contact when you're saying hi to people or listening. And speaking of listening, remember that the people who seem the most confident are not the people bragging about themselves. It's the people who ask questions and show interest in what others have to say!

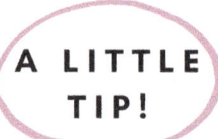 A LITTLE TIP!

HEALTH 101 | PAGE 42

HEY, LET'S TALK!

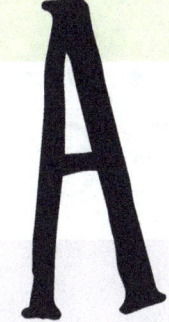LL THE DETAILS

USE THE FACT SHEET TO
COMPLETE THE BOXES BELOW.

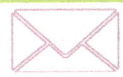 **TOPIC:** CONFIDENCE

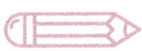 **THINGS TO REMEMBER:**

-
-
-
-
-

 I'M WONDERING:

-
-

 CHECK IN:

Confidence comes naturally.

a. true
b. false

HEALTH 101 | PAGE 43

HEY, LET'S TALK!

Big Differences

Let's explore male and female differences in a little more detail.

» HORMONES............................
✗ The primary hormone in a boy's body is not estrogen, like it is in your body. Their main hormone is **testosterone**. Testosterone causes puberty changes in their body that look completely different than yours!

» VOICE CHANGES....................
✗ Boys begin to get a deeper voice as they move through puberty. Their vocal cords thicken which gives off a lower sound.

» BIGGER..................................
✗ Because of testosterone, boys begin growing taller and bigger during puberty. You may notice their shoulders getting stronger looking and even their jaw lines becoming more pronounced.

» FACIAL HAIR..........................
✗ Boys will begin noticing hair growing in new areas of their body, just like you. But unlike you, they'll also begin seeing hair grow on their face. It might start off light and barely noticeable, but this hair will grow thicker with age and some boys choose to begin shaving their face.

What other similarities and differences do you notice or wonder about?

_____

_____

_____

HEY, LET'S TALK!

REMINDERS
Personal truths you must always remember!

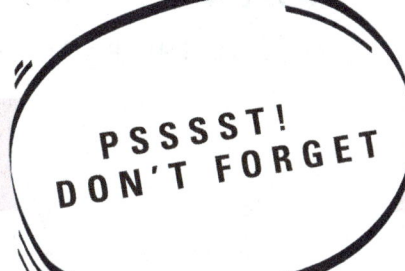

Our private parts are private.
That means that no one can look at, touch, or take pictures of this area.

We should always keep our hands to ourselves.
This means that we should never touch others' private parts, either.

Feelings and thoughts are normal.
Feelings of attraction for girls can rise up, but that doesn't have to control our actions or what we say and do.

Your body deserves to be safe.
If someone ever does touch you or make you feel uncomfortable, be sure to tell a trusted adult. Never keep a secret about this.

There are always adults you can trust.
Parents, teachers, pastors, coaches, and counselors often are people that can be trusted. Remember your personal list of "safe adults" on page 21.

HEY, LET'S TALK!

RATE YOUR UNDERSTANDING
COLOR THE FACE THAT SHOWS HOW WELL YOU UNDERSTAND EACH CONCEPT

Concept	I understand all of it	I understand most of it	I understand some of it
SHAVING + HAIR	🙂	😐	😠
ACNE + GROWING	🙂	😐	😠
BREASTS + BRAS	🙂	😐	😠
MOODS + SMELLING AWESOME	🙂	😐	😠
PERIODS + PERIOD SUPPLIES	🙂	😐	😠

HEALTH 101 | PAGE 46

HEY, LET'S TALK!

MYTH OR FACT?

LET'S SEE HOW MUCH YOU'VE **LEARNED** SINCE WE STARTED THIS WORKBOOK!

SITUATION	MYTH OR FACT?
Puberty looks the same for girls as it does for boys.	MYTH OR FACT
Everyone starts puberty at the same time.	MYTH OR FACT
Everyone has happy feelings about going through puberty.	MYTH OR FACT
Hormones are the cause of changes in puberty.	MYTH OR FACT
There are things you can do to slow down puberty.	MYTH OR FACT
People can always tell when you are going through puberty.	MYTH OR FACT
Your feelings and emotions can feel different during puberty.	MYTH OR FACT
Some parts of puberty can feel uncomfortable.	MYTH OR FACT
Puberty happens slowly, spanning a few years.	MYTH OR FACT
Puberty is an important part of your life.	MYTH OR FACT

HEY, LET'S TALK!

Times of Change

Let's explore what we notice, think, feel, and wonder about this time in life.

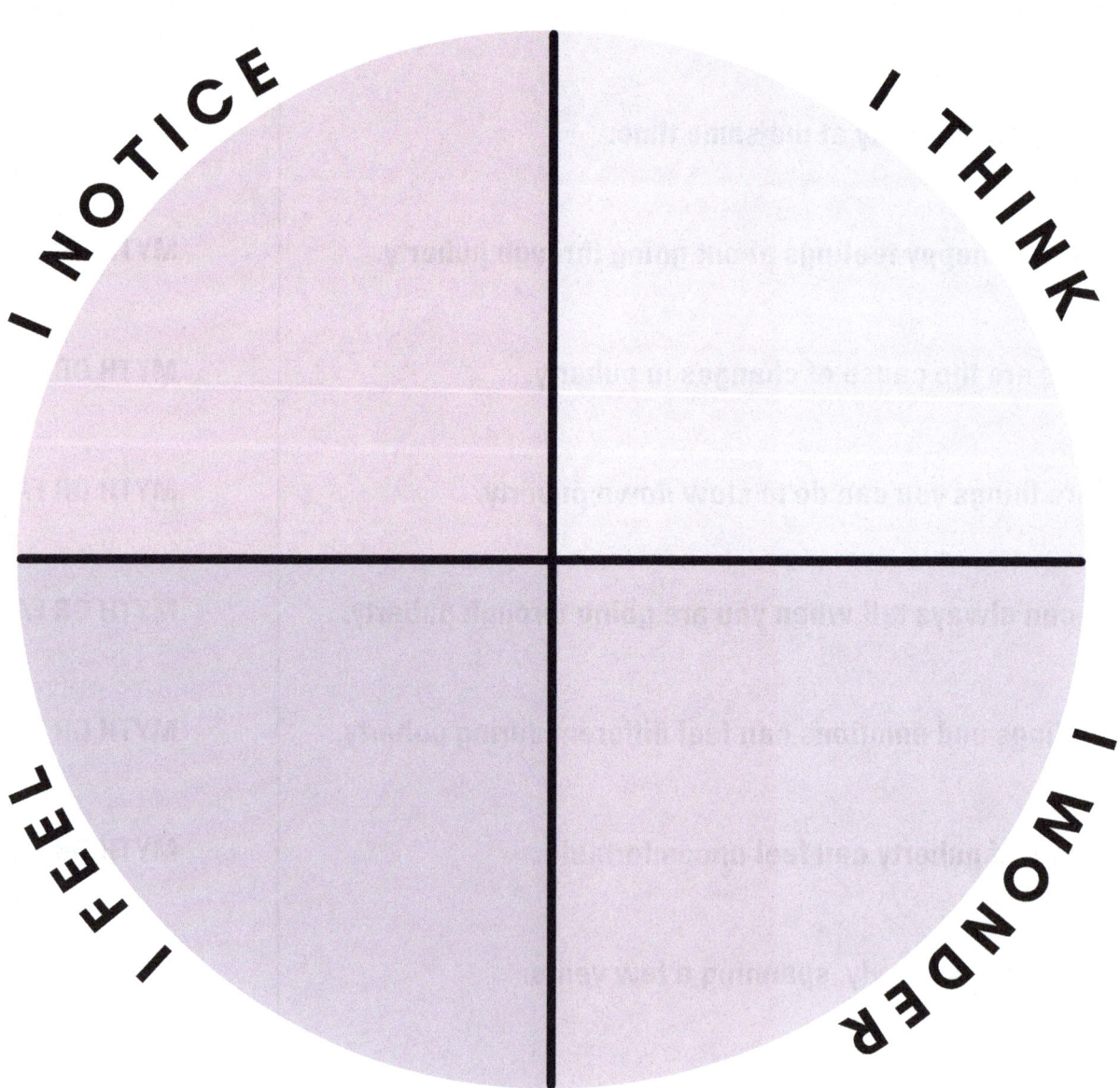

I NOTICE | I THINK | I FEEL | I WONDER

HEALTH 101 | PAGE 48

HEY, LET'S TALK!

WHAT WOULD YOU DO?

What could you **say**, **ask**, or **do** if you're stuck in any of the situations below?

Situation	
You get your **period** for the first time during the school day.	
A girl your age **brags** about how she is more grown up than you because she is further into puberty.	
You notice a friend is starting to **smell** lately every time you hang out.	
You really want to **shave** but you've never been shown how. You're not even sure if it's the right time yet.	
You start developing breasts and you're feeling **uncomfortable** about it.	

HEALTH 101 | PAGE 49

HEY, LET'S TALK!

PUBERTY + STRESS

Brainstorm some feelings or situations that feel stressful during this time of your life in each of the categories below.

HOME	
SCHOOL	
FRIENDS	
PERSONAL	
SOCIAL MEDIA	

HEY, LET'S TALK!

LIFE GOALS

Write your **goals** for each time of life in the triangle below.

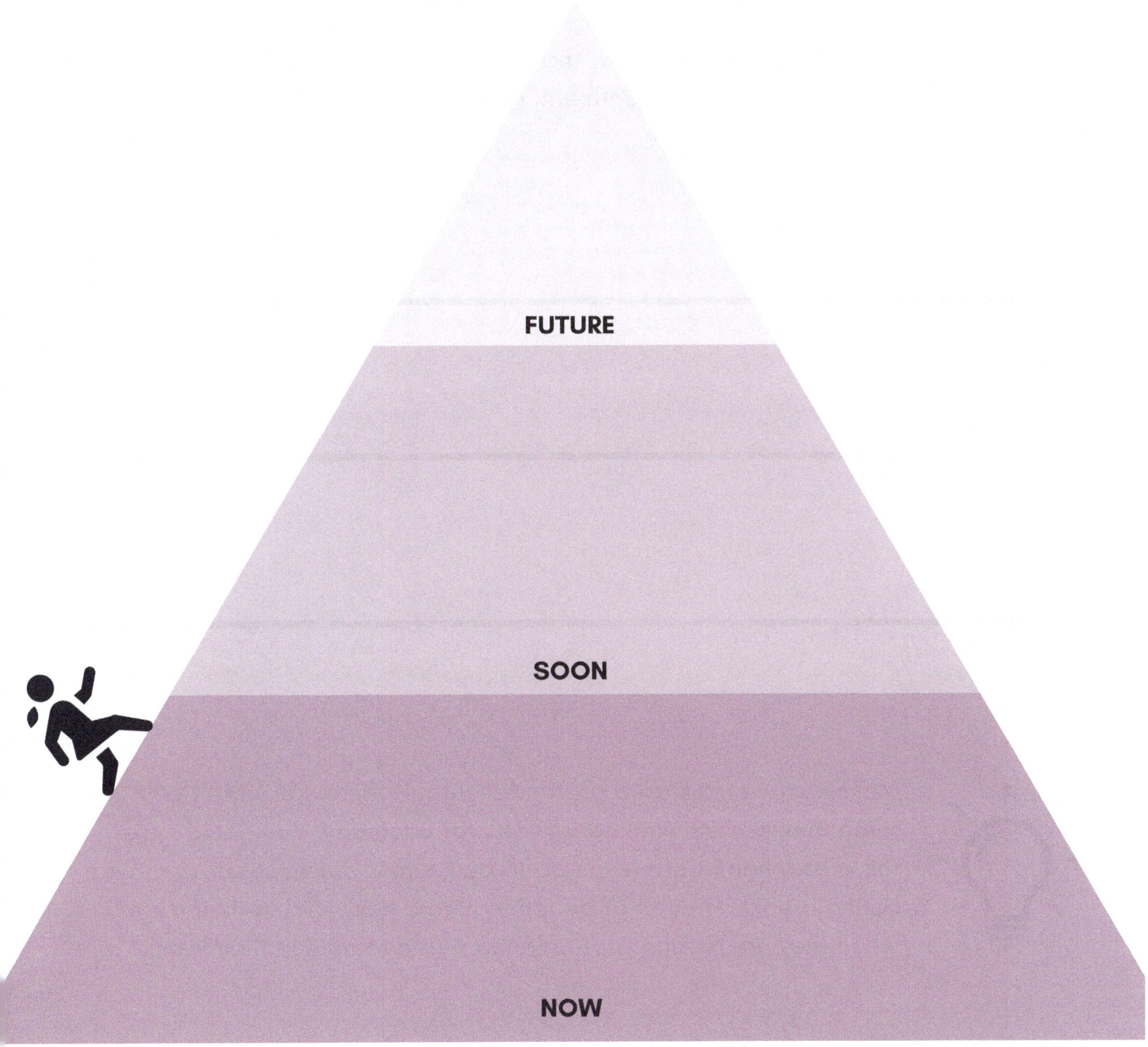

- FUTURE
- SOON
- NOW

HEY, LET'S TALK!

GRATITUDE

What are **3** things you are grateful for today?

Gratitude is **THANKFULNESS**! Studies show that practicing gratitude on a regular basis can increase feelings of happiness, contentment, and peace in your life.

_____

_____

3
_____

 Maybe you could start a gratitude journal where you write down three things which you are grateful for each day. You could make this a new habit before you go to bed, when you wake up, or maybe during breakfast. A lot of people notice a happy lift in their days when they are making gratitude journals a routine in their lives!

HEY, LET'S TALK!

ANONYMOUS QUESTIONS
Does it ever feel hard to ask a question about puberty?

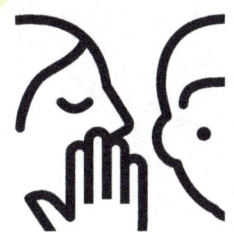

HERE'S AN IDEA FOR YOU!

Cut out a question strip from this workbook any time you want to ask a **question** but feel too uncomfortable asking it out loud.

Writing your question down and passing it on to an adult you trust is a way to ease the awkwardness.

QUESTION STRIPS!
USE THESE ANY TIME YOU WANT TO TALK WITH A GROWN UP YOU TRUST.

SOMETHING I'M WONDERING IS:

SOMETHING I'M WONDERING IS:

SOMETHING I'M WONDERING IS:

SOMETHING I'M WONDERING IS:

© 2021 EMILY KISZKA | HEALTH 101

HEY, LET'S TALK!

ANONYMOUS QUESTIONS
YOU CAN USE YOUR QUESTION STRIPS IN ANY WAY YOU'D LIKE!

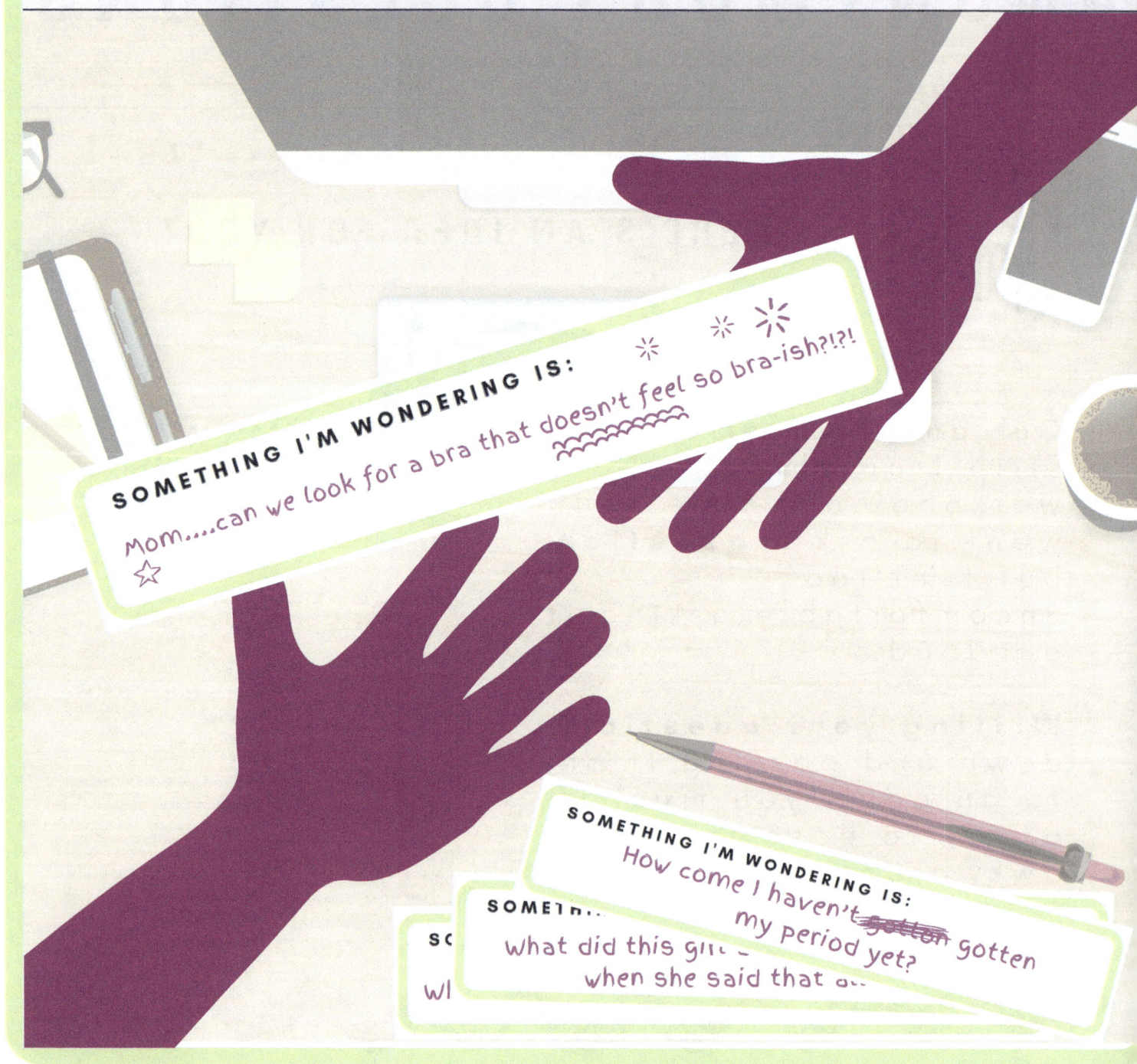

HEALTH 101 | ANONYMOUS QUESTIONS

HEY, LET'S TALK!

QUESTION STRIPS!
USE THESE ANY TIME YOU WANT TO WRITE A QUESTION TO A GROWN UP YOU TRUST.

SOMETHING I'M WONDERING IS:

SOMETHING I'M WONDERING IS:

SOMETHING I'M WONDERING IS:

SOMETHING I'M WONDERING IS:

HEALTH 101 | ANONYMOUS QUESTIONS

HEY, LET'S TALK!

SOMETHING I'M WONDERING IS:

✂ ― ― ― ― ― ― ― ― ― ― ― ― ― ―

SOMETHING I'M WONDERING IS:

― ― ― ― ― ― ― ― ― ― ― ― ― ― ―

SOMETHING I'M WONDERING IS:

― ― ― ― ― ― ― ― ― ― ― ― ― ― ―

SOMETHING I'M WONDERING IS:

― ― ― ― ― ― ― ― ― ― ― ― ― ― ―

SOMETHING I'M WONDERING IS:

HEALTH 101 | ANONYMOUS QUESTIONS

HEY, LET'S TALK!

SOMETHING I'M WONDERING IS:

✂ ---------------------------------

SOMETHING I'M WONDERING IS:

SOMETHING I'M WONDERING IS:

SOMETHING I'M WONDERING IS:

SOMETHING I'M WONDERING IS:

HEALTH 101 | ANONYMOUS QUESTIONS

HEY, LET'S TALK!

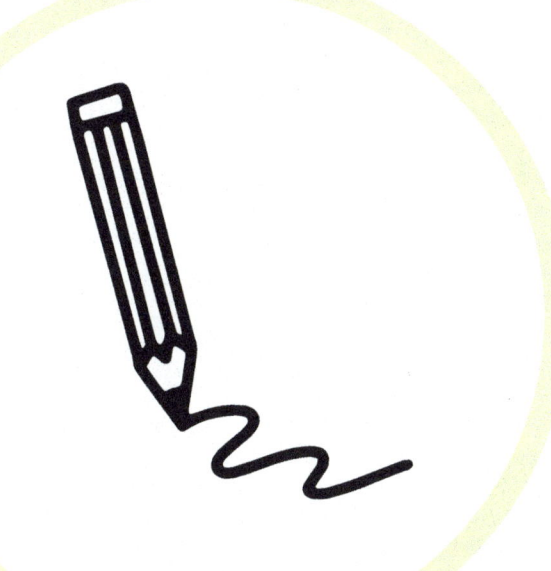

JOURNALING SPACE

HEY, LET'S TALK!

HEALTH 101 | JOURNAL PAPER

HEY, LET'S TALK!

HEALTH 101 | JOURNAL PAPER

HEY, LET'S TALK!

HEALTH 101 | JOURNAL PAPER

HEY, LET'S TALK!

HEALTH 101 | JOURNAL PAPER

HEY, LET'S TALK!

HEALTH 101 | JOURNAL PAPER

HEY, LET'S TALK!

HEALTH 101 | JOURNAL PAPER

HEY, LET'S TALK!

HEALTH 101 | JOURNAL PAPER

HEY, LET'S TALK!

APPENDIX
+
GLOSSARY

APPENDIX

PUBIC HAIR

HEY, LET'S TALK!

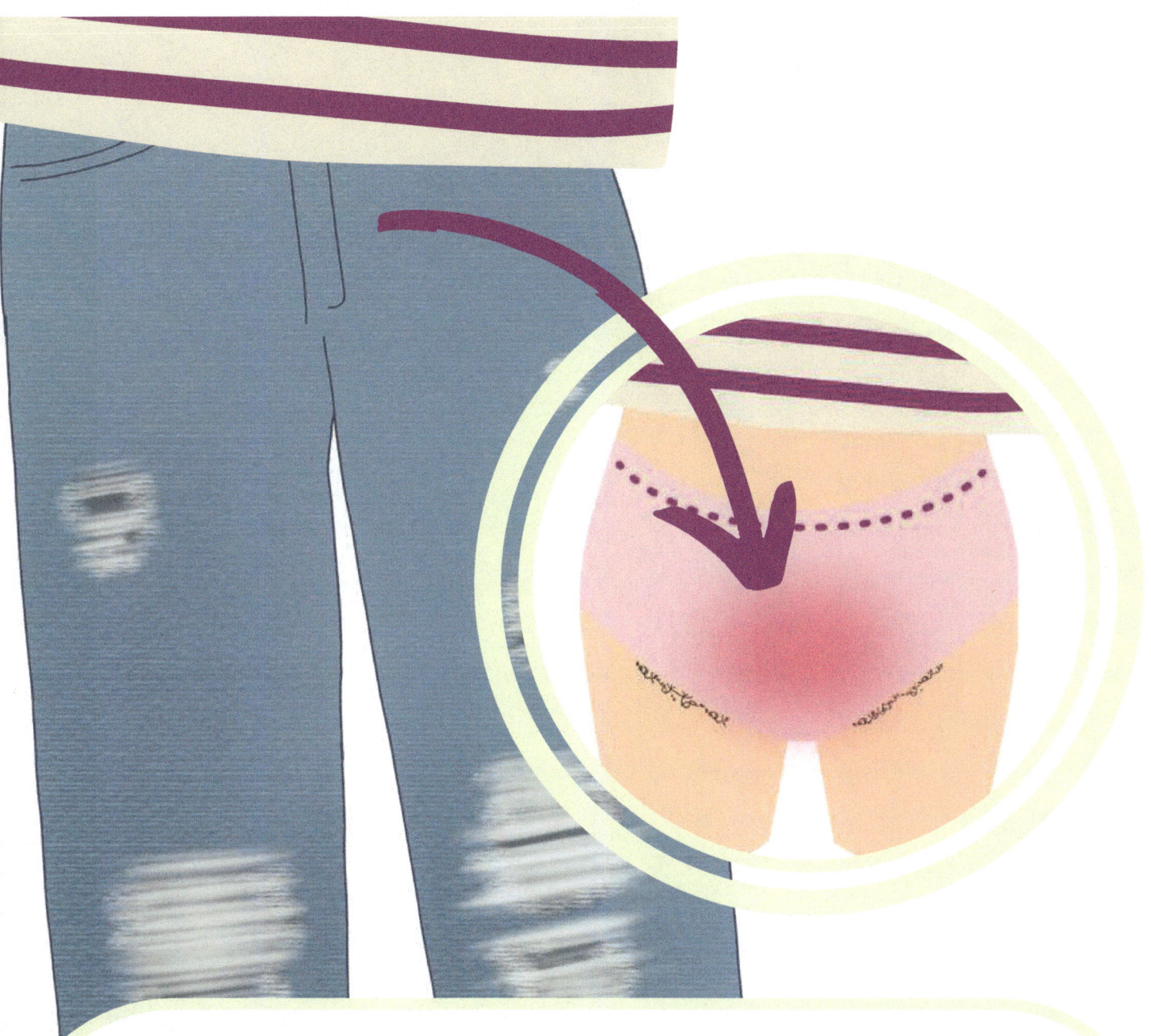

PUBIC HAIR
This shaded area highlights where the darker and coarser hair starts to grow on your body. Over time, it will spread toward the crease where your body and leg meet.

HEALTH 101 | APPENDIX A

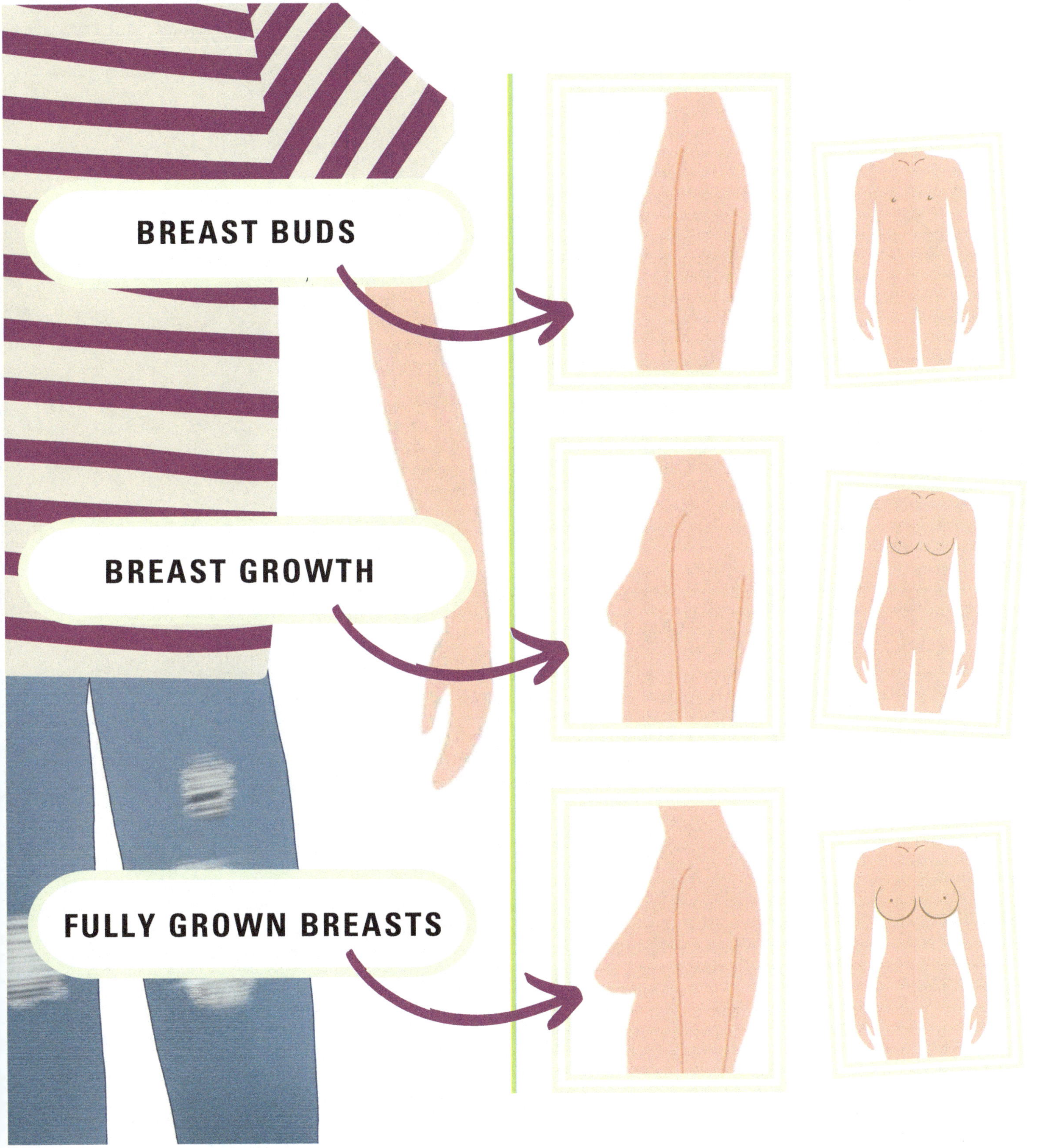

BREAST DEVELOPMENT

HEY, LET'S TALK!

- BREAST BUDS
- BREAST GROWTH
- FULLY GROWN BREASTS

HEALTH 101 | APPENDIX B

UTERUS, VAGINA　　　　　　　　　　　　　　　　　HEY, LET'S TALK!

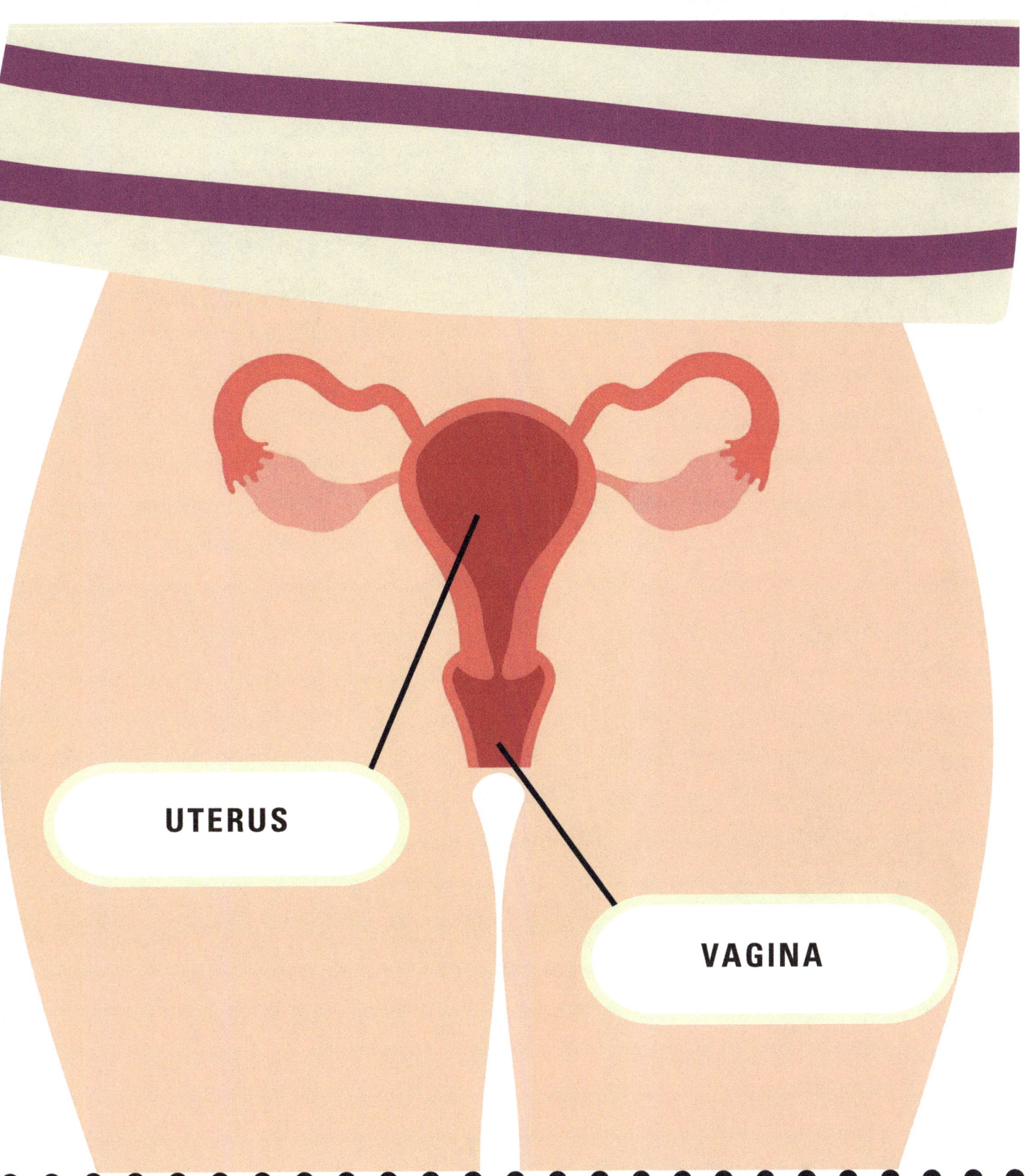

HEALTH 101 | APPENDIX C

VAGINA LOCATION HEY, LET'S TALK!

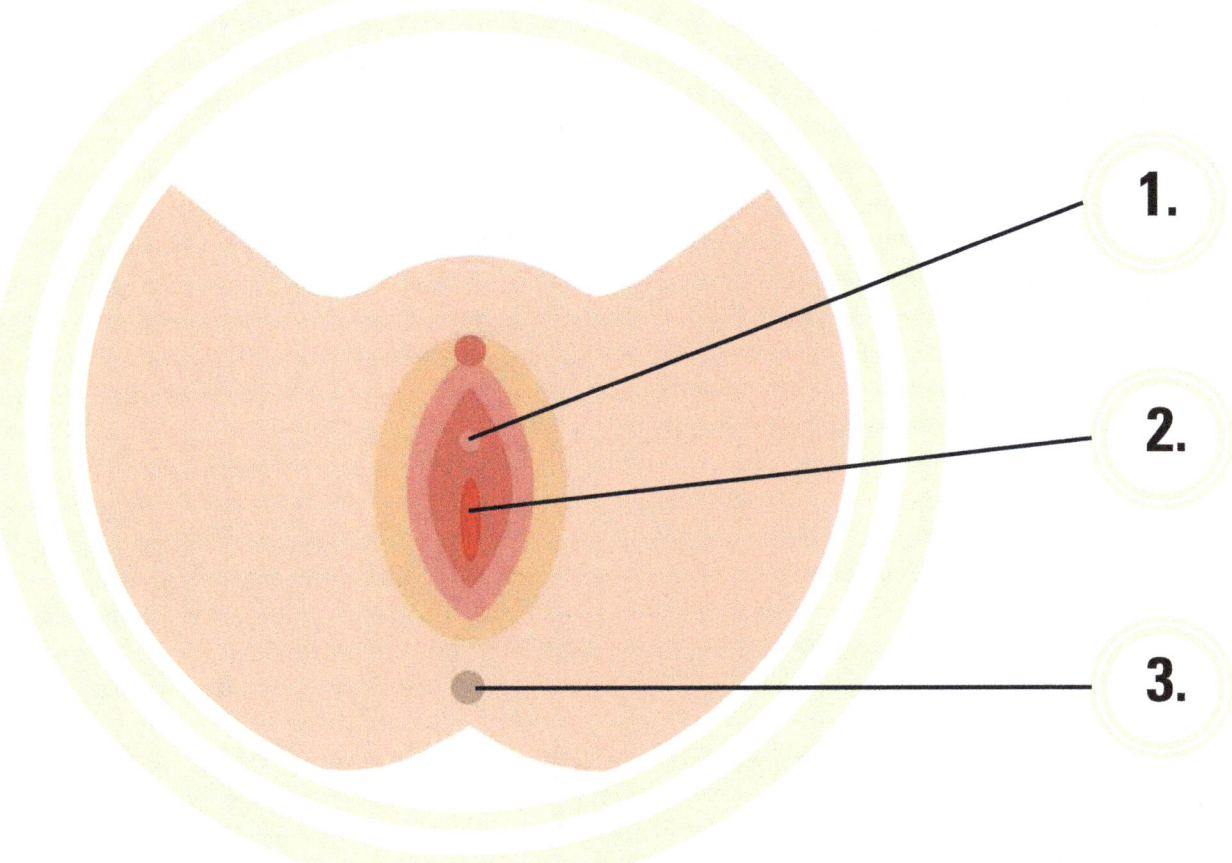

1. The Urethra
The Urethra is where urine (pee) leaves your body.

2. The Vagina
The Vagina is where blood leaves your body during your period and it is where the baby leaves the body during childbirth.

3. The Anus
The Anus is where feces (poop) leaves your body.

HEALTH 101 | APPENDIX D

PERIOD TRACKING　　　　　　　　　　　　　　　　HEY, LET'S TALK!

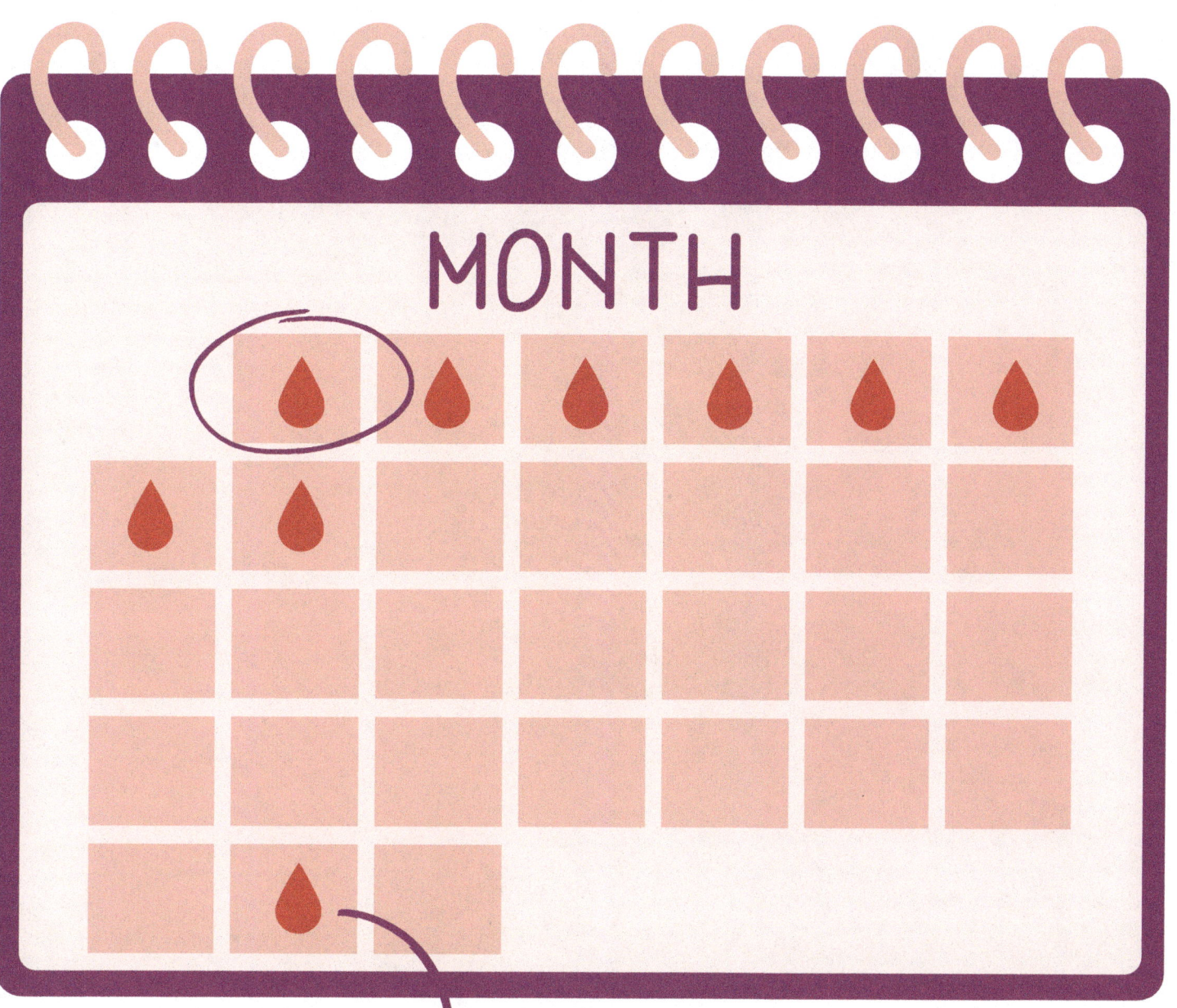

PERIOD TRACKING
You can estimate the start of each period by counting out four weeks from the first day of your last period.

HEY, LET'S TALK!

ACNE: Skin issues and irritations comprised of blackheads, whiteheads, and red pimples (or zits) that can surface on the face and also other areas of the body.

BREAST: A protuberance or rounded bump or mass, surmounted by a nipple, located on each side of the upper chest of a woman. Begins as a breast bud during puberty. Also commonly known as "Boobs."

BREAST BUD: A tiny mass under the nipple that is the beginning stage of breast development. Can be painful at times.

DISCHARGE: A slow release of fluid or mucous from the vagina noticeable at the start of puberty. A daily process that cleans the vagina.

ESTROGEN: A naturally occurring hormone that regulates development and body function in females.

HORMONES: Chemical substances that are secreted by the body internally into the bloodstream.

HYGIENE: Keeping the body and its surroundings clean to promote health.

MENSTRUAL PERIOD: A once-a-month flow of blood from the vagina. It is the shedding of the lining of the uterus and lasts for 4-7 days.

PERIOD: Also known as the Menstrual Period.

PUBERTY: A time of life where a child's body begins to change into an adult's body.

PUBIC HAIR: Coarse, dark hair that grows on the pubic region during and after puberty.

PRETEEN: A young person who is not yet a teenager; usually between the ages of 11-13.

TESTOSTERONE: The hormone that regulates development in males.

UTERUS: A female internal organ in which babies develop and are nourished until birth; also known as "the womb." Contains a lining which sheds during the Menstrual Cycle when the female is not pregnant.

VAGINA: The passageway or canal in a female that leads from the outside of the body to the uterus.

Made in United States
Orlando, FL
02 March 2025